Healthy Keto Bread Cookbook

Delicious and Low Carb Recipes
for Burning Fat and Losing Weight

Sarah James

TABLE OF CONTENTS

INTRODUCTION

Keto bread is a low-carbohydrate, high-fat liquid diet plan that requires you to consume a lot of healthy fats through either a keto bread recipe book or diet program. It's short for the controversial low-carbohydrate ketogenic diet more commonly referred to as the ketogenic diet. There are many variations of the keto diet with different levels of restrictions. For example, some people may only get 20 grams of carbohydrates per day while others restrict their intake to 5 grams of carbohydrates per day. The keto diet can be used as a short term diet, but most people choose to follow it for more than a month.

How Does Keto Bread Help You Lose Weight?

The idea behind the keto bread diet is that when you eat lots of healthy fats such as butter, olive oil, avocados, macadamia nuts, eggs, and grass-fed meats you will lose weight quickly and easily. The key to losing weight fast with this kind of eating plan is to take in so many calories through fat that you end up burning off the extra calories you burned from food intake. The keto bread diet plan isn't hard to follow if you stick to the rules. It's just a matter of cutting out most carbs and eating lots of healthy fats.

Is Eating Keto Bread Right For You?

If you want to lose weight fast and lose it completely with no chance of gaining it back then the keto bread recipe book or ketogenic diet might be right for you. It's not right for everyone though and can't be used in place of other methods like exercise and eating less food on your own as part of your weight loss program. If you're going to use this kind of eating plan make sure you check w/ your doctor first to see if it's right for you before putting it into action

The Keto diet has become more popular in the last few years. It is a low-carb, high-fat eating style that has been highly researched and proven to be effective. Here at Keto Bread, we have all of the necessary tools for anyone who is interested in changing their eating patterns to something healthier, such as the Men's Standard Keto Cookbook.

We understand that everyone's nutritional needs are different, so we have cataloged a wide variety of recipes to meet your needs. Keto is a deficient carbohydrate diet with ample protein, which is allowed during the diet. It is not just a ketogenic change in the diet and grows healthy eating habits. They create healthy and natural eating habits for you stronger both physically and mentally. Our body needs energy as it is coming from carbohydrates; our body uses glucose (carbohydrates) as a primary energy source.

The ketogenic diet is a low-calorie, high-fat diet in which fat is converted into energy instead of glucose. During this process, fatty acids are released from your body, and our liver renovates these fatty acids into ketones. When ketone levels have increased in the blood goes to the brain and replaces glucose with energy. You can reach this stage in the first week of the ketogenic diet.

The keto diet is not new, but its popularity has declined over time as various medical developments seem to help with conditions like epilepsy and weight loss. However, now, people are again beginning to see it as a way to lose weight, lighten skin, maintain their health, and even live longer. So much to wait for!

Our body uses glucose as its primary source of energy. Never Carbohydrates are metabolized, and glucose is produced in our body. This glucose is stored in the cells of our body. When glucose levels rise, then the excess glucose is converted to glycogen. This chemical process of the conversion of glucose to glycogen is called glycogenesis. This glycogen is stored in the muscles of the body and liver as a backup source of energy. In this diet, your body undergoes many adjustments. Some different signs and symptoms confirm that you are in ketosis.

BASIC BREAD

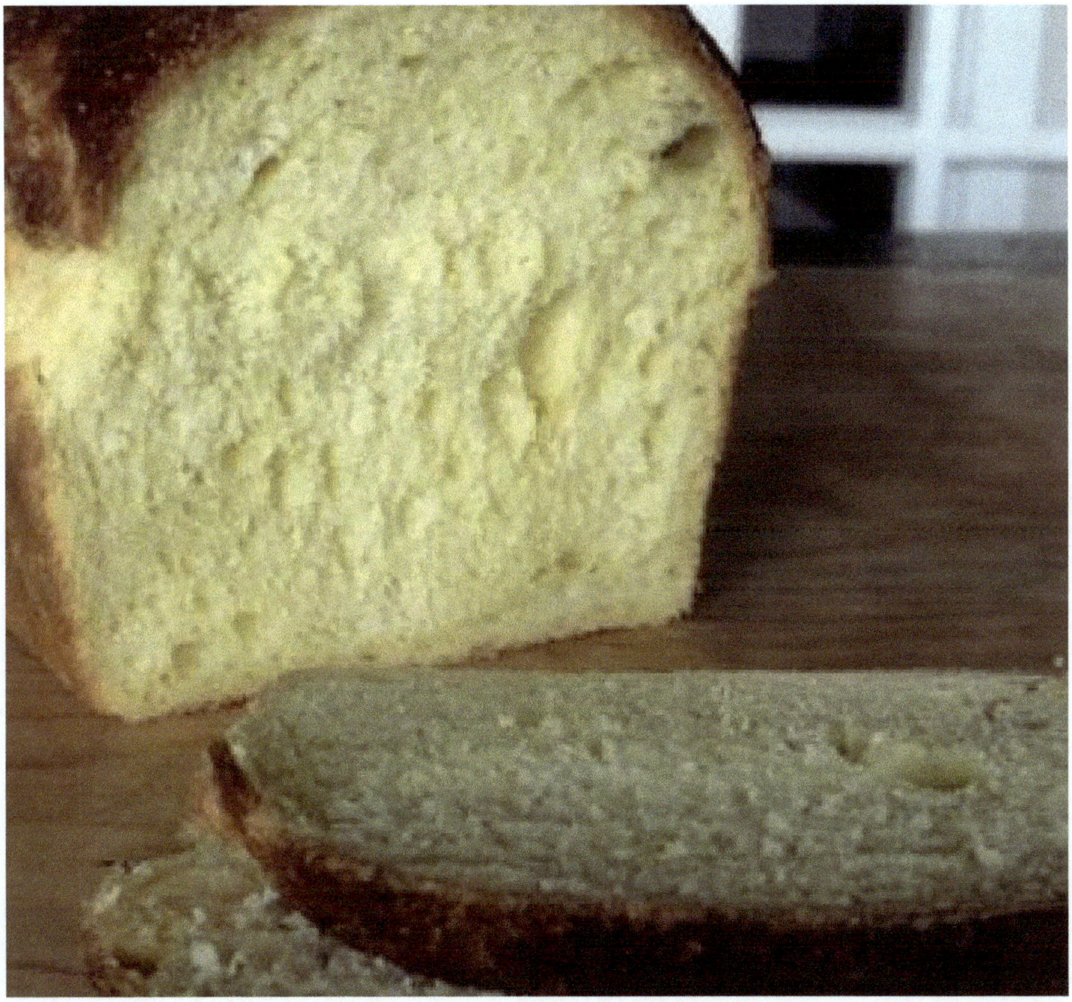

KETO BLUEBERRY-BANANA LOAF

Preparation time: 10 minutes

Cooking time: 2 hours 20 minutes

Servings: 12 slices

Ingredients:

½ cup warm water

1 tablespoon almond milk, unsweetened

2 eggs, small

8 tablespoons butter, melted, and unsalted

3 medium-sized mashed bananas

0.75 teaspoon stevia extract

2 cups almond flour

½ teaspoon salt

2 teaspoons baking powder

1 teaspoon baking soda

1 cup frozen blueberries

Directions:

Prepare the ingredients. Beat the eggs and mash the bananas.

Soften the butter in the microwave for 30 seconds. Mix the water and the milk.

Put the bananas, eggs, butter, water, and milk in the bread bucket.

Add in all dry ingredients except blueberries. Start the bread machine by selecting Quick Bread, then close the lid. After the first kneading, open the lid and add in the blueberries.

Close the lid and let the cycle continue until the end. Once cooked, remove the bread from the bucket and let it cool in a cooling rack before slicing. Serve.

Nutrition:

Calories: 119 | Calories from Fats: 90 | Total Fats: 9 g | Total Carbohydrates: 9 g
Net Carbohydrates: 7 g | Proteins: 2 g

ANISE ALMOND BREAD

Preparation time: 10 minutes

Cooking time: 3 hours

Servings: 1 loaf

Ingredients:

3/4 cup water

1 or 1/4 cup egg substitute

1/4 cup butter or margarine, softened

1/4 cup sugar - 1/2 teaspoon salt

3 cups bread flour

1 teaspoon anise seed

2 teaspoons active dry yeast

1/2 cup almonds, chopped small

Directions:

Add all ingredients to machine pan except almonds.

Select Basic bread setting. After prompt, add almonds.

Nutrition:

Calories: 78 | Total Fats: 4 g | Carbs: 7 g | Fibers: 0 | Proteins: 3 g

THREE INGREDIENT BUTTERMILK CORNBREAD

Preparation time: 10 minutes

Cooking time: 20 minutes

Servings: 8

Ingredients:

Vegetable oil as needed

1 and 1/2 cups buttermilk

1 and 1/2 cups cornmeal

1/2 cup all-purpose flour

Directions:

Preheat oven to 450 °F (230 °C). Pour enough oil into a skillet to coat the bottom; place into the oven.

Mix buttermilk, cornmeal, and flour together in a bowl until smooth.

Remove skillet from oven; pour in buttermilk mixture.

Bake in the preheated oven until cornbread is golden brown— 20 to 25 minutes.

Nutrition:

Calories: 157 | Total Fats: 2.6 g | Total Carbohydrates: 28.6 g

THE BEST CORN BREAD YOU'LL EVER EAT

Preparation time: 5 minutes

Cooking time: 30 minutes

Servings: 8

Ingredients:

1 egg

1 and 1/3 cups milk

1/4 cup vegetable oil

2 cups self-rising corn meal mix

1 (8 ounce) can cream-style corn

1 cup sour cream

Directions:

Heat oven to 425 °F (220 °C). Grease a 9 inch iron skillet.

In a large bowl, beat the egg.

Add milk, oil, sour cream, cream corn, and cornmeal mix; stir until cornmeal is just dampened.

Pour batter into greased skillet.

Bake for 25 to 30 minutes, or until knife inserted in center comes out clean.

Nutrition:

Calories: 328 | Total Fats: 15.9 g | Total Carbohydrates: 40.8 g | Proteins: 6.4 g

MACADAMIA NUT BREAD

Preparation time: 10 minutes

Cooking time: 40 minutes

Servings: 6

Ingredients:

5 oz. macadamia nuts

5 large eggs

¼ cup coconut flour

½ teaspoon baking soda

½ teaspoon apple cider vinegar

Directions:

Start by preheating the oven to 350 °F.

Blend macadamia nuts in a food processor until it forms a nut butter.

Continue blending while adding eggs one by one until well incorporated.

Stir in apple cider vinegar, baking soda, and coconut flour.

Blend until well mixed and incorporated.

Grease a bread pan with cooking spray and spread the batter in a pan.

Bake the batter for 40 minutes approximately until golden brown.

Slice and serve.

Nutrition:

Calories: 248 | Total Fats: 19.3 g | Saturated Fats: 4.8 g | Total Carbs: 3.1 g
Fibers: 0.6 g | Proteins: 7.9 g

BULGUR BREAD

Preparation time: 3 hours

Cooking time: 3 hours

Servings: 8

Ingredients:

½ cup bulgur

1/3 cup boiling water

1 egg - 1 cup water

1 tablespoon butter

1 ½ tablespoon milk powder

1 tablespoon sugar

2 teaspoons salt

3 ¼ cups flour

1 teaspoon dried yeast

Directions:

Pour bulgur in boiling water into a small container and cover with a lid.

Leave to stand for 30 min. Cut butter into small cubes.

Stir the egg with water in a measuring container. The total volume of eggs with water should be 300 ml.

Put all the ingredients in the bread maker in the order that is described in the instructions for your bread maker.

Bake in the Basic mode, Medium crust.

Nutrition:

Carbohydrates 3 g | Fats 3 g | Proteins 8.9 g | Calories 255 | Fibers 1.2 g

FRENCH HAM BREAD

Preparation time: 3 hours and 30 minutes

Cooking time: 3 hours and 30 minutes

Servings: 8

Ingredients:

3 and 1/3 cups almond flour

1 cup ham

½ cup milk powder

1 ½ tablespoons sugar

1 teaspoon yeast, fresh

1 teaspoon salt

1 teaspoon dried basil

1 and 1/3 cups water

2 tablespoons olive oil

Directions:

Cut ham into cubes of 0.5-1 cm (approximately ¼ inch).

Put the ingredients in the bread maker in the following order: water, olive oil, salt, sugar, flour, milk powder, ham, and yeast.

Put all the ingredients according to the instructions to your bread maker.

Put basil in a dispenser or fill it later at the signal in the container.

Turn on the bread machine. After the end of the Baking cycle, leave the bread container in the bread maker to keep warm for 1 hour.

Then your delicious bread is ready!

Nutrition:

Carbohydrates: 2 g | Fats: 5.5 g | Proteins: 11.4 g | Calories: 287 | Fibers: 1 g

SOURDOUGH KETO BAGUETTES

Preparation time: 5 minutes | Cooking time: 17 minutes | Servings: 10

Ingredients:

Dry Ingredients: 1/2 cup almond flour | 1/3 cup phylum husk powder | 1 teaspoon salt

1/2 cup coconut flour | 1/2 stuffed cup flax supper | 1 teaspoon preparing pop

Wet Ingredients: 6 large egg whites | 2 large eggs | 1 cup tepid water

3/4 cup low-fat buttermilk full-fat would make them excessively overwhelming and they may not rise | 1/4 cup white wine vinegar or apple juice vinegar

Directions:

Preheat the broiler to 180 °C/360 °F (fan helped). Use a kitchen scale to gauge every one of the ingredients cautiously. Blend all the dry ingredients in a bowl (almond flour, coconut flour, ground flaxseed, psyllium powder, heating pop, and salt).

In a different bowl, blend the eggs, egg whites, and buttermilk. The explanation you shouldn't use just entire eggs is that the bread wouldn't rise with such a large number of egg yolks in. Try not to squander them —use them for making Homemade Mayo, Easy Hollandaise Sauce, or Lemon Curd. For a similar explanation, use low-fat (not full-fat) buttermilk.

Add the egg blend and mix them well, using a blender until the mixture is thick. Add vinegar and tepid water and follow procedure until well combined. Don't over-process the mixture.

Using a spoon, make 8 ordinary or 16 smaller than usual rolls and place them on a preparing plate fixed with material paper or a non-stick tangle. They will rise, so make a point to leave some space between them. Alternatively, score the loaves slantingly and make 3-4 cuts.

Place in the stove and cook for 10 minutes. Then, decrease the temperature to 150 °C/300 °F and heat for another 30-45 minutes (little loaves will set aside because they need less effort to cook).

Remove from the stove, let the plate chill off and place the rolls on a rack to chill off to room temperature. Store them at room temperature on the off chance that you intend to use them in the following couple of days or store in the cooler for as long as 3 months.

Cooked products that use psyllium consistently result in a marginally wet surface. If necessary, cut the rolls down the middle and place in a toaster or in the broiler before serving.

Tip: To spare time, blend all the dry ingredients ahead and store in a zip-lock sack, and add a mark with the number of servings. At the point when fit to be prepared, simply include the wet ingredients!

Nutrition: Calories: 21 | Fats: 4.7 g | Carbs: 44.2 g | Proteins: 0 g | Sugar: 5 g

TOAST BREAD

Preparation time: 3 ½ hours

Cooking time: 3 ½ hours

Servings: 8

Ingredients:

1 ½ teaspoon yeast

3 cups almond flour

2 tablespoons sugar

1 teaspoon salt

1 ½ tablespoon butter

1 cup water

Directions:

Pour water into the bowl; add salt, sugar, soft butter, flour, and yeast.
(I add dried tomatoes and paprika)

Put it on the Basic program. The crust can be Light or medium.

Nutrition:

Carbohydrates 5 g | Fats 2.7 g | Proteins 5.2 g | Calories 203 | Fibers 1 g

WHOLE WHEAT BREAD

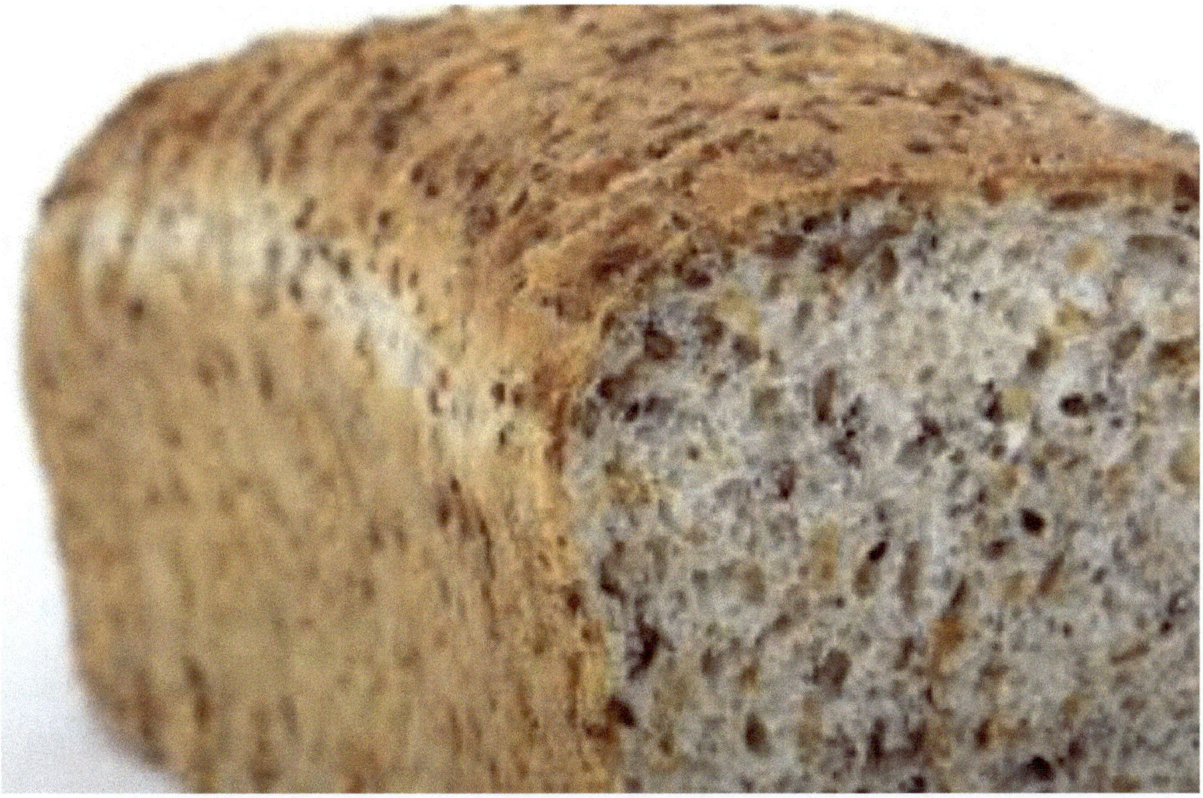

CRUNCHY HONEY WHEAT BREAD

Preparation Time: 7 minutes

Cooking Time: 3 hours and 30 minutes

Servings: 12 slices

Ingredients:

2 cups warm water at 1100°F (450°C)

2 tbsp. vegetable oil

1 tbsp. honey

½ tsp salt

1 cup bread flour

¼ cup whole wheat flour

1 tbsp. granola

Active dry yeast

Directions:

Place the ingredients into the bread machine following the order recommended by the manufacturer.

Choose the Whole Wheat setting or the Dough cycle on the machine.

Press the START button. Once the machine has finished the whole cycle of baking the bread in the oven, form the dough and add it into a loaf pan that's greased.

Let it rise in volume in a warm place until it becomes double its size.

Insert into the preheated 350°F (175°C) oven and bake for 35-45 minutes. Enjoy!

Nutrition:

Calories: 199 | Carbs: 37 g | Fats: 4.2 g | Proteins: 6.2 g

EASY HOME BASE WHEAT BREAD

Preparation Time: 10 minutes

Cooking Time: 3 hours and 50 minutes

Servings: 12 slices

Ingredients:

2 cups whole wheat flour

¼ cup bread flour

1 tbsp. butter softened

1 cup warm water at 900°F (320°C)

1 cup warm milk at 900°F (320°C)

Active dry yeast

2 eggs, at room temperature

½ tsp salt | 2 tbsp. honey

Directions:

Add the ingredients into the pan of the bread machine following the order suggested by the manufacturer.

Use the Whole Wheat cycle, choose the crust color, weight, and START the machine.

Check how the dough is kneading after five minutes pass because you may need to add either one tbsp. of water or one tbsp. of flour-based on consistency.

When the bread is complete, cool it on a wire rack before slicing. Enjoy!

Nutrition:

Calories: 180 | Carbs: 33 g | Fats: 2 g | Proteins: 7 g

WHOLE WHEAT YOGURT BREAD

Preparation Time: 10 minutes

Cooking Time: 3 hours and 40 minutes

Servings: 12 slices

Ingredients:

1 tbsp. ground nutmeg (optional)

2 cups water

2 tbsp. butter, melted

¼ cup plain yogurt

2 tbsp. dry milk

2 tbsp. honey

1 tbsp. active dry yeast

1 cup whole wheat flour

1 cup bread flour

2 tbsp. ground cinnamon

½ tsp salt

Directions:

Begin by pouring ingredients into the bread pan in the instruction your manufacturer endorses. In my case, liquids always go first. So, I begin with water, yogurt, butter, honey, sieve flour, dry milk, add salt, ground cinnamon, and yeast in different corners of the pan.

Select the Whole grain setting, light or medium crust, and press START. When ready, allow it to cool and then serve. Enjoy!

Nutrition:

Calories: 158 | Carbs: 20 g | Fats: 5 g | Proteins: 6 g

CHEESE BREAD

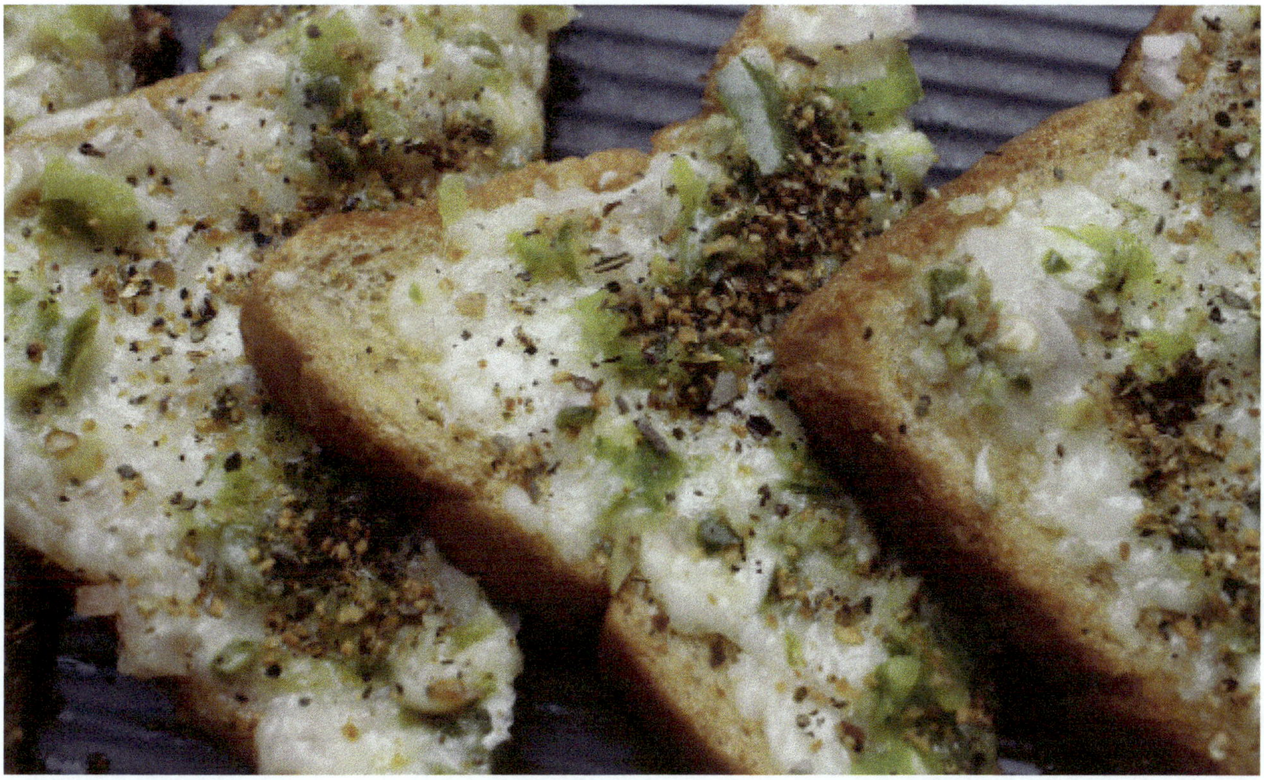

BEER AND CHEESE BREAD

Preparation Time: 10 minutes

Cooking Time: 25 minutes

Servings: 8

Ingredients:

3 cups bread or all-purpose flour

1 tbsp. instant yeast

1 tsp. salt 1 tbsp. sugar

1 and 1/2 cup beer at room temperature

1/2 cup shredded Monterey cheese

1/2 cup shredded Edam cheese

Directions:

Place all elements, except cheeses, in the bread pan in the liquid-dry-yeast layering.

Put the pan in the Zojirushi bread machine.

Select the Bake cycle.

Choose Regular Basic Setting. Press Start.

When the kneading process is about to end, add the cheese.

Wait until the loaf is cooked.

The machine will start the keep warm mode after the bread is complete.

Do not forget to let it stay in that mode for about 10 minutes before unplugging.

Lastly, remove the pan and let it cool down for about 10 minutes.

Nutrition:

Calories 174 | Carbs 31.1 g | Fats 3.1 g | Proteins 5.1 g

BLUE CHEESE ONION BREAD

Preparation Time: 10 minutes

Cooking Time: 25 minutes

Servings: 8

Ingredients:

1 ¼ cup water, at 80°F to 90°F

1 egg, at room temperature

1 tablespoon melted butter cooled

¼ cup powdered skim milk

1 tablespoon sugar

¾ teaspoon salt

½ cup (2 ounces) crumbled blue cheese

1 tablespoon dried onion flake

3 cups white bread flour

¼ cup instant mashed potato flakes

1 teaspoon bread machine or active dry yeast

Directions:

Preparing the Ingredients. Place the ingredients in your Zojirushi bread machine.

Program the machine for Regular Basic, select light or medium crust, and press Start.

Remove the bucket from the machine. Let the loaf cool for 5 minutes.

Gently shake the container to remove the loaf and turn it out onto a rack to cool.

Nutrition:

Calories 174 | Carbs 31.1 g | Fats 3.1 g | Proteins 5.1 g

CHEESE LOAF

Preparation Time: 10 minutes

Cooking Time: 25 minutes

Servings: 8

Ingredients:

1/4 cup flour

1 tsp. instant yeast

1 and 3/4 cup water

1 tbsp. sugar

1 and 1/2 cup shredded cheddar cheese

1 tbsp. parmesan cheese

1 tsp. mustard

1 tsp. paprika

1 tbsp. minced white onion

1/3 cup butter

Directions:

Begin through placing all ingredients in the bread pan in the liquid-dry-yeast layering.

Put the pan in the Zojirushi bread machine. Select the Bake cycle.

Choose Regular Basic Setting and light crust. Press start and wait until the loaf is cooked.

The machine will start the keep warm mode after the bread is complete.

For about 10 minutes, let the bread stay for 10 minutes in that mode before unplugging.

You may now want to remove the pan and let it cool down for about 10 minutes.

Nutrition:

Calories 174 | Carbs 31.1 g | Fats 3.1 g | Proteins 5.1 g

SPICE AND HERB BREAD

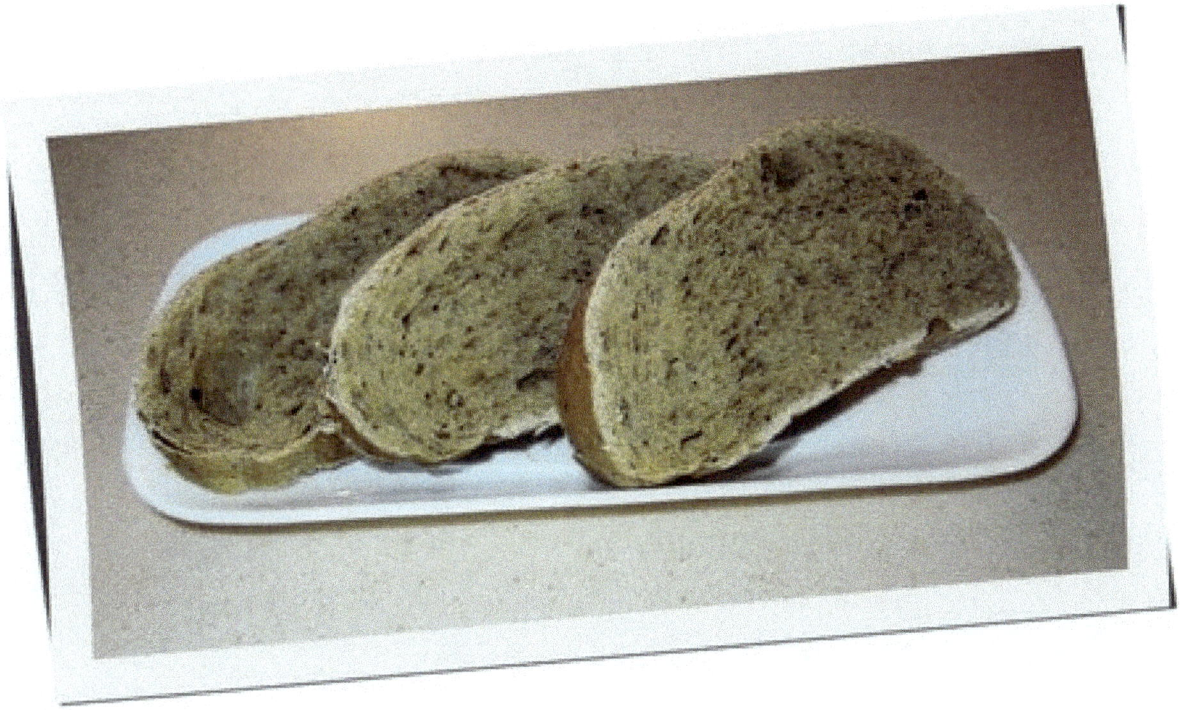

ROSEMARY BREAD

Preparation Time: 2 hours and 40 minutes

Cooking Time: 25-30 minutes

Servings: 1 loaf

Ingredients:

1 cup water

2 tablespoons olive oil

1 and 1/2 teaspoon white sugar

1 and 1/2 teaspoon salt

1/4 teaspoon Italian seasoning

1/4 teaspoon ground black pepper

1 tablespoon dried rosemary

1/2 cup bread flour

1 and 1/2 teaspoon active dry yeast

Directions:

Into the bread machine pan, put the ingredients following the order recommended by manufacturer.

Use the white bread cycle and then push the Start button.

Nutrition:

Calories: 137 | Total Carbohydrates: 21.6 g | Cholesterol: 0 mg | Total Fats: 3.9 g
Proteins: 3.6 g | Sodium: 292 mg

SAFFRON TOMATO BREAD

Preparation Time: 3 hours and 30 minutes

Cooking Time: 15 minutes

Servings: 10

Ingredients:

1 teaspoon bread machine yeast

2 ½ cups wheat bread machine flour

1 tablespoon panifarin

1 ½ teaspoon kosher salt

1 ½ tablespoon white sugar

1 tablespoon extra-virgin olive oil

1 tablespoon tomatoes, dried and chopped

1 tablespoon tomato paste

½ cup firm cheese (cubes)

½ cup feta cheese | 1 pinch saffron | 1 ½ cup serum

Directions:

Five minutes before cooking, pour in dried tomatoes and 1 tablespoon of olive oil.

Add the tomato paste and mix. Place all the dry and liquid ingredients, except additives, in the pan and follow the instructions for your bread machine.

Pay particular attention to measuring the ingredients. Use a measuring cup, measuring spoon, and kitchen scales to do so.

Set the baking program to BASIC and the crust type to MEDIUM. Add the additives after the beep or place them in the dispenser of the bread machine.

Shake the loaf out of the pan. If necessary, use a spatula.

Wrap the bread with a kitchen towel and set it aside for an hour. Otherwise, you can cool it on a wire rack.

Nutrition: Calories: 260 | Total Carbohydrates: 35.5 g | Cholesterol: 20 g | Sugar: 5.2 g Total Fats: 9.2 g | Proteins: 8.9 g | Sodium: 611 mg

CRACKED BLACK PEPPER BREAD

Preparation Time: 3 hours 30 minutes

Cooking Time: 15 minutes

Servings: 8

Ingredients:

¾ cup water, at 80°F to 90°F

1 tablespoon melted butter, cooled

1 tablespoon sugar

¾ teaspoon salt

2 tablespoons skim milk powder

1 tablespoon minced chives

½ teaspoon garlic powder

½ teaspoon cracked black pepper

2 cups white bread flour

¾ teaspoon bread machine or instant yeast

Directions:

Place the ingredients in your bread machine as recommended by the manufacturer.

Program the machine for Basic/White bread, select light or medium crust, and press Start. When the loaf is done, remove the bucket from the machine.

Let the loaf cool for 5 minutes. Gently shake the bucket to remove the loaf, and turn it out onto a rack to cool.

Nutrition:

Calories: 141 | Total Carbohydrates: 27 g | Total Fats: 2 g | Proteins: 4 g | Fibers: 1 g Sodium: 215 mg

SPICY CAJUN BREAD

Preparation Time: 2 hours

Cooking Time: 15 minutes

Servings: 8

Ingredients:

¾ cup water, at 80°F to 90°F

1 tablespoon melted butter, cooled

2 teaspoons tomato paste

1 tablespoon sugar

1 teaspoon salt

2 tablespoons skim milk powder

½ tablespoon cajun seasoning

1/8 teaspoon onion powder

2 cups white bread flour

1 teaspoon bread machine or instant yeast

Directions:

Place the ingredients in your bread machine as recommended by the manufacturer.

Program the machine for Basic/White bread, select light or medium crust, and press Start. When the loaf is done, remove the bucket from the machine.

Let the loaf cool for 5 minutes. Gently shake the bucket to remove the loaf, and turn it out onto a rack to cool.

Nutrition:

Calories: 141 | Total Carbohydrates: 27 g | Total Fats: 2 g | Proteins: 4 g | Fibers: 1 g Sodium: 215 mg

ANISE LEMON BREAD

Preparation Time: 2 hours

Cooking Time: 15 minutes

Servings: 8

Ingredients:

2/3 cup water, at 80°F to 90°F

1 egg, at room temperature

2 and 2/3 tablespoons butter, melted and cooled

2 and 2/3 tablespoons honey

1/3 teaspoon salt

2/3 teaspoon anise seed

2/3 teaspoon lemon zest

2 cups white bread flour

1 and 1/3 teaspoons bread machine or instant yeast

Directions:

Place the ingredients in your bread machine as recommended by the manufacturer.

Program the machine for Basic/White bread, select light or medium crust, and press Start. When the loaf is done, remove the bucket from the machine.

Let the loaf cool for 5 minutes. Gently shake the bucket to remove the loaf, and turn it out onto a rack to cool.

Nutrition:

Calories: 158 | Total Carbohydrates: 27 g | Total Fats: 5 g | Proteins: 4 g | Fiber: 1 g Sodium: 131 mg

CARDAMON BREAD

Preparation Time: 2 hours

Cooking Time: 15 minutes

Servings: 8

Ingredients:

½ cup milk, at 80°F to 90°F

1 egg, at room temperature

1 teaspoon melted butter, cooled

2 teaspoons honey

2/3 teaspoon salt

2/3 teaspoon ground cardamom

2 cups white bread flour

¾ teaspoon bread machine or instant yeast

Directions:

Place the ingredients in your bread machine as recommended by the manufacturer.

Program the machine for Basic/White bread, select light or medium crust, and press Start. When the loaf is done, remove the bucket from the machine.

Let the loaf cool for 5 minutes. Gently shake the bucket to remove the loaf, and turn it out onto a rack to cool.

Nutrition:

Calories: 149 | Total Carbohydrates: 29 g | Total Fats: 2g | Proteins: 5 g | Fiber: 1 g Sodium: 211 mg

VEGETABLE BREAD

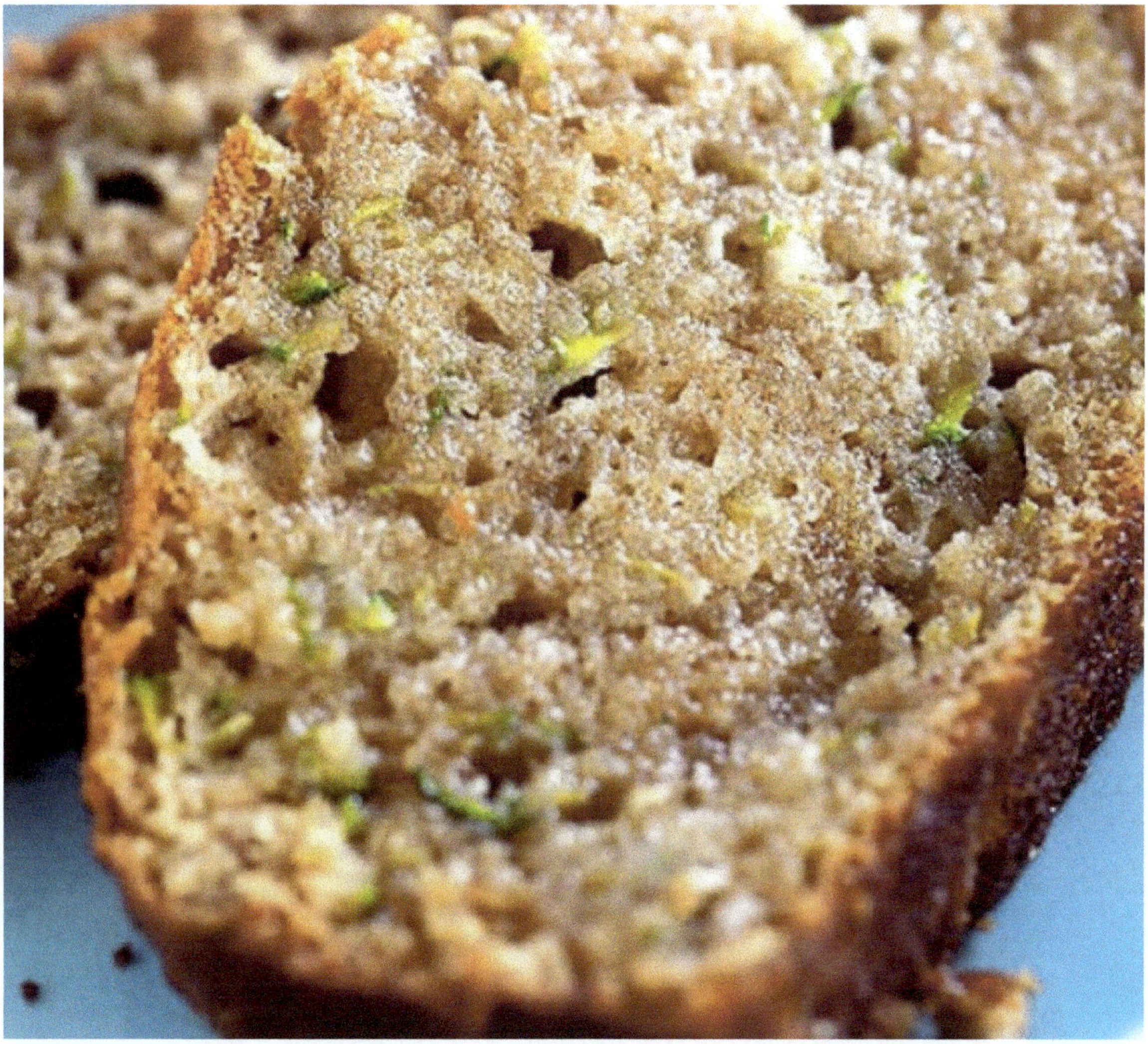

TOMATO BREAD

Preparation time: 15 minutes

Cooking Time: ¾ hour

Servings: 1.5 Lb. / 16 Slices

Ingredients:

4 whole eggs | ¼ tsp sea salt

2 tbsp. salted butter, melted

1 cup flaxseed meal | 4 tsp. oat fiber

¼ tsp. garlic powder | 2 tsp. keto baking powder

1 ½ tsp. xanthan gum | ½ tsp. dried basil

¼ cup parmesan, grated

2 tbsp. sun-dried tomatoes, diced

Directions:

Prepare all of the ingredients for your bread and gather your measuring tools (a cup, a spoon, kitchen scales). Carefully whisk eggs and butter together.

Pour all the ingredients into the bread machine pan. Close the cover.

Set your bread machine program to CAKE for 30 – 45 minutes (depending on the bread machine model) and choose the crust color LIGHT. Press START.

Help the bread machine knead the dough with a spatula, if necessary.

Before the baking mode begins, sprinkle the top with grated parmesan. After baking for 20 minutes, check for doneness with a toothpick. Wait until the program is complete.

When done, take the bucket out and let it cool for 5-10 minutes. Shake the loaf from the pan and let cool for 30 minutes on a cooling rack.

Slice, serve with a soup or a salad, and enjoy the taste of fragrant homemade keto bread.

Nutrition: Calories 88 | Net Carbs 0.6 g | Total Fats 6.1 g | Saturated Fats 2.4 g | Cholesterol 48 g Sodium 243 mg | Total Carbohydrates 2.6 g

HEARTY CHEESY BROCCOLI BREAD

Preparation time: 35 minutes

Cooking Time: 30 minutes

Servings: 4

Ingredients:

5 eggs, whisked

2 teaspoons baking powder

1 cup cheddar, shredded

1 cup broccoli florets, separated

4 tablespoons coconut flour

Cooking spray

Directions:

In a bowl, mix all the ingredients except the cooking spray and stir the batter really well.

Pour batter in the bread machine pan pre-greased with cooking spray.

Set the bread machine to the basic bread setting.

When the bread is done, remove bread machine pan from the bread machine.

Let cool slightly before transferring to a cooling rack.

Cool the bread down, slice / serve.

Nutrition:

Calories 123 | Fats 6 g | Fibers 1 g | Carbs 3 g | Proteins 6 g

HOT RED PEPPER BREAD

Preparation time: 15 minutes

Cooking Time: 1 hour

Servings: 12

Ingredients:

2 cups of dried, roasted hot red peppers, crushed

2 tsp. of active dry yeast

1 tsp. of pepper powder | 2 eggs

2 tsp. of warm water

½ cup of unsweetened almond milk

Salt, half a teaspoon | 1 ½ tsp. of baking powder

Almond flour, two cups | Coconut flour, one cup

Melted unsalted butter, two teaspoons

Directions:

Get a mixing container and combine the almond flour, dried and crushed roasted hot red peppers, salt, coconut flour, and baking powder.

Get another mixing container and combine the eggs, unsweetened almond milk, warm water, and melted unsalted butter.

As per the instructions on the manual of your machine, pour the ingredients in the bread pan, following the instructions of adding the yeast.

Place the bread pan in the machine, and select the sweet bread setting, together with the bread size and crust type, if available, then press start once you have closed the lid of the machine.

When the bread is ready, extract it, and place it on a metallic mesh surface to cool completely before cutting and eating it.

Nutrition:

Calories 107 | Fats 5.45 g | Fibers 1.8 g | Carbs 7.86 g | Proteins 8.22 g

HERBED KETO BREAD

Preparation time: 5 minutes

Cooking Time: 40 minutes

Servings: 8

Ingredients:

3 cups coconut flour

1 teaspoon baking powder

1 teaspoon baking soda

2 teaspoons stevia

1 ½ cup warm water

½ teaspoon basil, dried

1 teaspoon oregano, dried

½ teaspoon thyme, dried

½ teaspoon marjoram, dried

2 tablespoons olive oil

Directions:

In a bowl, mix the flour with baking powder, baking soda, stevia, basil, oregano, thyme, and the marjoram and stir.

Add the rest of the ingredients, stir well and transfer the dough in the bread machine loaf pan pre-greased with cooking spray. However, take a look to the manufacturer's instructions for mixing dry and wet ingredients.

Place the bread pan in the machine, and select the basic bread setting, together with the bread size, if available, then press start once you have closed the lid of the machine.

When the bread is ready, using oven mitts, remove the bread pan from the machine.

Cool the bread down before serving.

Nutrition: Calories 200 | Fats 7 g | Fibers 3 g | Carbs 5 g | Proteins 6 g

LIGHT CORNBREAD

Preparation time: 15 minutes

Cooking Time: 40 minutes

Servings: 8

Ingredients:

Eggs, 4

Almond flour, 1 and a half cup full

Swerve Keto sweetener half a cup

Extract of vanilla, 1 teaspoon

Baking powder, 1 teaspoon

Unsalted melted butter, 4 teaspoons

Directions:

Prepare a mixing container, where you will combine the almond flour, Swerve sweetener, and baking powder.

In another mixing container, combine the eggs, pure vanilla extract, and unsalted melted butter. As per the instructions on the manual of your machine, pour the ingredients in the bread pan, taking care to follow how to mix in the yeast.

Place the bread pan in the machine, and select the basic bread setting, together with the bread size and crust type, if available, then press start once you have closed the lid of the machine.

When the bread is ready, using oven mitts, remove the bread pan from the machine.

Use a stainless spatula to extract the bread from the pan, and turn the pan upside down on a metallic rack where the bread will cool off before slicing it.

Nutrition:

Calories 66 | Fats 1.78 g | Fibers 0.1 g | Carbs 11 g | Proteins 1.16 g

ZUCCHINI LEMON BREAD

Preparation time: 5 minutes

Cooking Time: 40 minutes

Servings: 12

Ingredients:

2 cups of almond flour

Salt, 3/4 teaspoon

Baking powder, 1 teaspoon

Baking soda, half a teaspoon

Zucchini grated; 2 cups full

Extract of vanilla, 2 teaspoons

Swerve sweetener, a third cup

Zest from 2 lemons | 3 eggs

Melted butter, unsalted, three-quarters of a cup full

Juice of a fresh lemon, 2 teaspoons

Active dry yeast, 1 and a half teaspoon

Directions:

In a mixing container, combine the almond flour, salt, baking powder, and baking soda.

Get another mixing bowl and combine the shredded zucchini, pure vanilla extract, lemon zest, lemon juice, eggs, and unsalted melted butter.

As per the instructions on the manual of your machine, pour the ingredients in the bread pan, taking care to follow how to mix in the yeast.

Place the bread pan in the machine, and select the basic bread setting, together with the bread size and crust type, if available, then press start once you have closed the lid of the machine.

When the bread is ready, using oven mitts, remove the bread pan from the machine.

Use a stainless spatula to extract the bread from the pan and turn the pan upside down on a metallic rack where the bread will cool off before slicing it.

Nutrition:

Calories 230 | Fats 17.98 g | Fibers 0.2 g | Carbs 15.23 g | Proteins 2.58 g

ONION BREAD

Preparation time: 20 minutes

Cooking time: 5 minutes

Servings: 6

Ingredients:

1 red onion diced and sautéed with ½ tsp. of butter until golden brown

3 tsp. of melted unsalted butter

Salt, a quarter teaspoon

Ground garlic, a quarter teaspoon

Psyllium husk flour, 3 teaspoons

5 eggs | Baking powder, half a teaspoon

Active dry yeast, three-quarters of a teaspoon

Onion powder, half a teaspoon | Almond flour, 1 cup

Directions:

Get a mixing container and combine the almond flour, salt, psyllium husk flour, ground onion, baking powder, and ground garlic.

Get another mixing container and mix the melted unsalted butter, eggs, and sautéed onions. As per the instructions on the manual of your machine, pour the ingredients in the bread pan, also following the instructions for the yeast.

Place the bread pan in the machine, and select the basic bread setting, together with the bread size and crust type, if available, then press start once you have closed the lid of the machine.

When the bread is ready, extract it, and place it on a metallic mesh surface to cool completely before cutting and eating it.

Nutrition:

Calories 127 | Fats 9.48 g | Fiber 0.3 g | Carbs 2.07 g | Proteins 7.97 g

SWEET BREAD

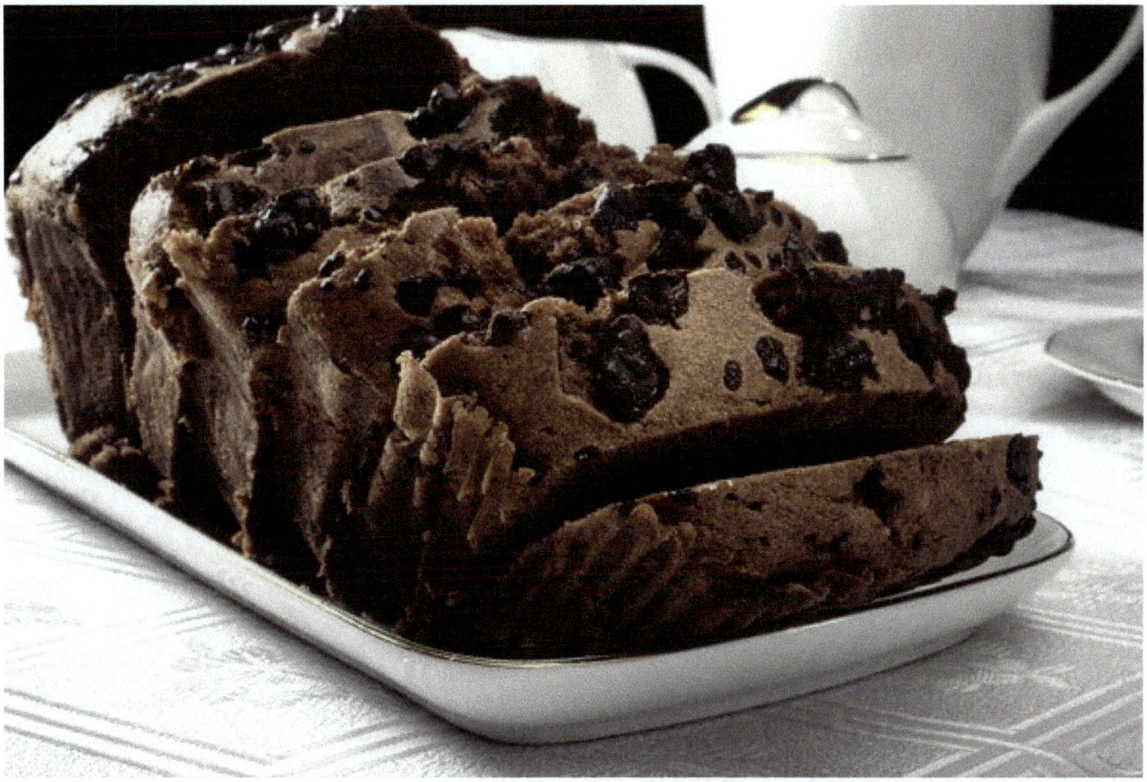

DELICIOUS CARROT CAKE

Preparation time: 15 minutes

Cooking time: 55 minutes

Servings: 6

Ingredients:

2 large eggs | ½ cup carrots, grated

1 teaspoon vanilla | 3 tablespoons heavy cream

2 tablespoons coconut oil, melted

¼ teaspoon nutmeg | ½ teaspoon cinnamon

1 teaspoon baking powder | 2/3 cup swerve | 1 cup almond flour

For Frosting: 1 tablespoon heavy cream

½ teaspoon vanilla | 2 teaspoons fresh lemon juice

3 tablespoons swerve | 4 ounces cream cheese, softened

Directions:

Take a cake pan which fits into the instant pot, spray with cooking spray and set aside.

Drain excess liquid from grated carrots. In a mixing bowl, mix together almond flour, grated carrots, vanilla, coconut oil, heavy cream, eggs, nutmeg, cinnamon, baking powder, and swerve using a hand mixer until well combined.

Pour batter into the prepared cake pan and cover the pan with foil. Add 1 2/3 cup of water to the instant pot, then place steamer rack into the pot.

Place cake pan on the steamer rack. Seal the instant pot with the lid and select manual high pressure and set the timer for 45 minutes.

Allow releasing pressure naturally for 10 minutes, then release using the Quick release method. Open the lid carefully and remove the cake pan from the pot.

Let the cake cool for 30 minutes. Meanwhile, make the frosting. In a large bowl, add heavy cream, vanilla, lemon juice, swerve, and cream cheese and beat using a hand mixer until creamy.

Once the cake is cool completely, then frost the cake using prepared cream.

Cut cake into slices and serve.

Nutrition: Calories: 289 | Fats: 25.9 g | Carbohydrates: 10.9 g | Proteins: 7.9 g

PURPLE YAM PANCAKES

Preparation time: 5 minutes

Cooking time: 10 minutes

Servings: 4

Ingredients:

½ cup coconut flour

4 eggs

1 cup coconut milk

1 teaspoon guar gum

½ teaspoon baking powder

1 tablespoon coconut oil

¼ cup purple yam puree

Directions:

Mix all ingredients in a blender.

Preheat a skillet and coat with non-stick spray.

Ladle in the batter and cook for 1-2 minutes per side.

Nutrition:

Kcal per serve: 347 | Fats: 31 g (76%) | Proteins: 11 g (13%) | Carbs: 9 g (11%)

ALMOND COCONUT CAKE

Preparation time: 10 minutes

Cooking time: 50 minutes

Servings: 8

Ingredients:

2 eggs, lightly beaten

½ cup heavy cream

¼ cup coconut oil, melted

1 teaspoon cinnamon

1 teaspoon baking powder

1/3 cup swerve

½ cup unsweetened shredded coconut

1 cup almond flour

Directions:

Spray a 6-inch cake pan with cooking spray and set aside. In a large bowl, mix together the almond flour, cinnamon, baking powder, swerve, and shredded coconut.

Add eggs, heavy cream, and coconut oil into the almond flour mixture and mix until well combined. Pour batter into the prepared cake pan and cover the pan with foil.

Add 2 cups of water into the instant pot, then place a steamer rack in the pot.

Place cake pan on top of steamer rack. Seal the instant pot with the lid and select manual high pressure and set the timer for 40 minutes.

Once the timer goes off, allow to release pressure naturally for 10 minutes and then release using Quick-release method. Open the lid carefully.

Remove the cake pan from the pot and let it cool for 20 minutes.

Cut cake into slices and serve.

Nutrition: Calories: 228 | Fats 21.7 g | Carbohydrates: 5.2 g | Proteins: 5 g

TASTY CHOCOLATE CAKE

Preparation time: 10 minutes

Cooking time: 30 minutes

Servings: 6

Ingredients:

3 large eggs

¼ cup butter, melted

1/3 cup heavy cream

1 teaspoon baking powder

¼ cup walnuts, chopped

¼ cup unsweetened cocoa powder

2/3 cup swerve

1 cup almond flour

Directions:

Spray cake pan with cooking spray and set aside. Add all ingredients into a large mixing bowl and mix using a hand mixer until the mixture looks fluffy.

Pour batter into the prepared cake pan. Pour 2 cups of water into the instant pot, then place a steamer rack in the pot. Place cake pan on top of steamer rack.

Seal the instant pot with the lid and cook on manual high pressure for 20 minutes.

Allow releasing pressure naturally for 10 minutes, then release using the Quick release method. Open the lid carefully.

Remove the cake pan from the pot and let it cool for 20 minutes.

Cut cake into slices and serve.

Nutrition:

Calories 275 | Fats 25.5 g | Carbohydrates: 7.5 g

LEMON CHEESECAKE

Preparation time: 10 minutes

Cooking time: 35 minutes

Servings: 8

Ingredients:

For crust: 2 tablespoons coconut oil, melted

2 tablespoons swerve | ¾ cup almond flour | pinch of salt

For filling: 2 tablespoons heavy whipping cream

2 large eggs | 1 teaspoon lemon extract

1 teaspoon lemon zest | 4 tablespoons fresh lemon juice

2/3 cup swerve | 1 lb. cream cheese, softened

Directions:

Grease a 7-inch spring-form pan with butter and line with parchment paper. Set aside.

In a bowl, combine together all the crust ingredients and pour into the prepared pan and spread evenly, and place in the refrigerator for 15 minutes.

In a large mixing bowl, beat cream cheese using a hand mixer until smooth.

Add swerve, lemon extract, lemon zest, and lemon juice and beat again until just combined. Add eggs and heavy whipping cream and beat until well combined.

Pour the filling mixture over the crust and spread evenly. Cover the springform pan with foil. Pour 1 cup of water into the instant pot, then place a trivet in the pot.

Place cake pan on top of the trivet. Seal instant pot with the lid and select manual high pressure for 35 minutes. Allow releasing pressure naturally, then open the lid.

Remove the cake pan from the pot and let it cool completely.

Place in refrigerator for 3-4 hours. Serve chilled and enjoy.

Nutrition:

Calories: 322 | Fats: 31.1 g | Carbohydrates: 4.4 g | Proteins: 8.3 g

SAVORY BREAD

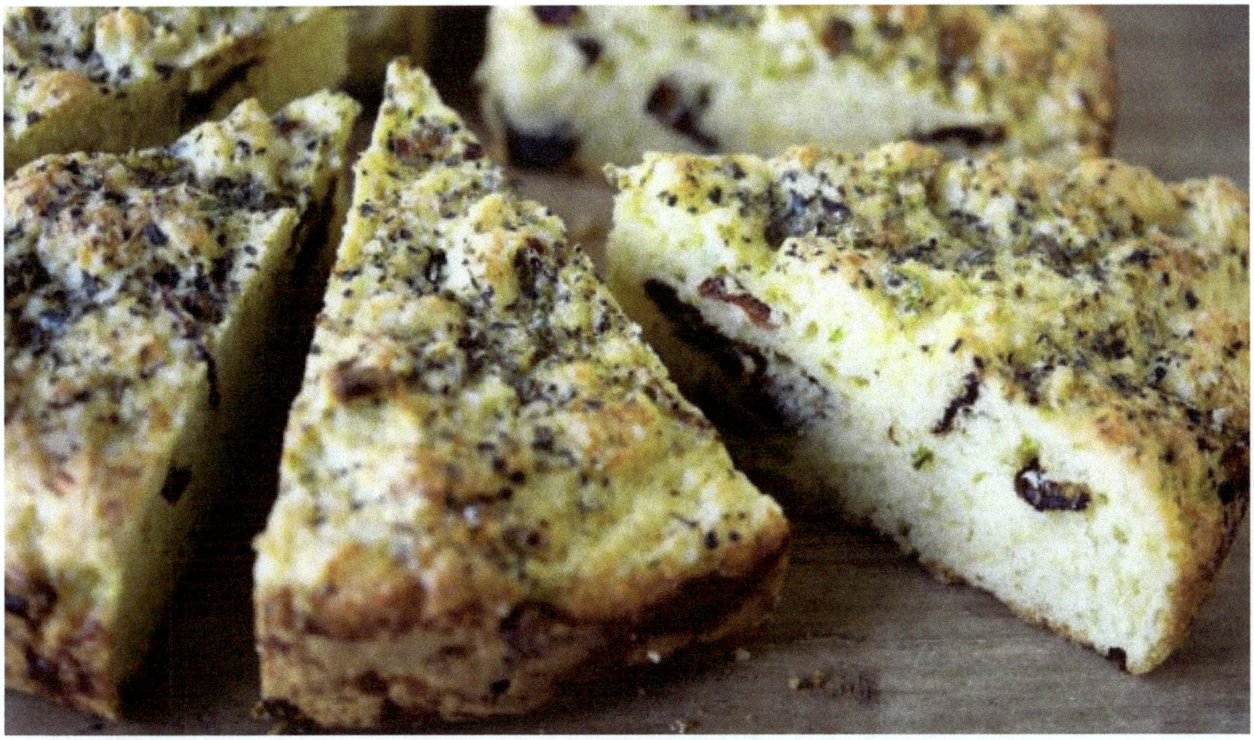

EASY BLENDER FLATBREAD WITH A TOUCH OF CINNAMON

Preparation time: 5 minutes

Cooking time: 14 minutes

Servings: 4

Ingredients:

Cream cheese - 2 oz.

Eggs - 2

Protein powder - 1 scoop

Cinnamon - a pinch

Coconut oil - 1 tablespoon

Salt - a pinch

Directions:

Take a blender and blend in the cream cheese, eggs, protein powder, cinnamon and the salt.

Heat up a frying pan with coconut oil and put in the batter to fry.

Cook the flatbread on both sides.

Serve when done!

Nutrition:

Calories: 163 | Fats: 13.26 g | Carbs: 2.41 g | Proteins: 8.67 g

LOW CARB VANILLA BREAD

Preparation time: 10 minutes

Cooking time: 30 minutes

Servings: 5

Ingredients:

Eggs, separated - 5

Coconut flour - 4tbsp

Granulated sweetener - 4tbsp

Baking powder - 1tsp

Vanilla extract - 2tsp

Full fat milk - 3tbsp

Melted butter - 125 grams

Directions:

Separate the egg whites and the egg yolks and beat the egg whites until they form in to stiff peaks. In another bowl, beat the egg yolks, coconut flour, granulated sweetener and the baking powder.

Now slowly and gradually pour in the melted butter carefully and mix it to make sure that you have a very smooth consistency of your batter.

Now add in the full fat milk and the vanilla extract.

With the help of a rubber spatula, now very gently fold in the egg whites in the mixture.

Try to keep as much as air and fluffiness that you can for better results.

Preheat your oven at 350 degrees Fahrenheit and put the pan to bake in preheated oven for 30 minutes or until it is golden brown.

Cool and then serve!

Nutrition:

Calories: 175 | Fats: 9.89 g | Carbs: 10.51 g | Proteins: 9.37 g

VERY YUMMY CHOCOLATE BREAD

Preparation time: 5 minutes

Cooking time: 15 minutes

Servings: 1

Ingredients:

Cocoa powder - 2 tablespoons

Almond flour - ½ cup

Erythritol - 2 tablespoons

Egg - 1

Heavy cream - 1 tablespoon

Vanilla extract - ½ teaspoon

Baking powder - ¼ teaspoon

Salt - a pinch

Directions:

Preheat your oven at 350 degrees Fahrenheit. Whisk together the cocoa powder, almond flour and the sweetener erythritol and make sure to remove lumps.

In another bowl, beat the egg well. Now add the egg, heavy cream and the vanilla extract in to the erythritol mixture and mix. Add in the salt and baking powder as well.

Mix all the ingredients properly. Grease your pan, pour the batter in and then put it to bake in preheated oven for 10 to 15 minutes or until the bread is done.

Serve while the bread cool down.

Nutrition:

Calories: 139 | Fats: 11.55 g | Carbs: 1.55 g | Proteins: 7.1 g

WHOLE GRAIN BREAD

Preparation time: 10 minutes

Cooking time: 40-45 minutes

Servings: 6

Ingredients:

Eggs - 2 | Flour - ¼ cup

Skim milk - 1 ¾ cup

Canola oil - ¼ cup

Applesauce - ¼ cup

Vanilla extract - 1 teaspoon

Pastry flour - 1 cup

Flax seed meal - ½ cup

Wheat germ - ¼ cup

Baking powder - 4 teaspoons

Sugar - 1 tablespoon

Salt - ¼ teaspoon

Directions:

Preheat your oven at 350 degrees Fahrenheit.

In a bowl, first mix the wet ingredients such as the eggs, skim milk, canola oil, applesauce, vanilla extract with the dry ones that are pastry flour, flax seed meal and the wheat germ.

Now mix in the flour, baking powder, sugar and salt.

Pour the batter in to the prepared pan and bake until the bread turns golden brown.

Cool and serve!

Nutrition:

Calories: 234 | Fats: 13.9 g | Carbs: 19.41 g | Proteins: 7.98 g

CHEDDAR AND CHIVE BREAD

Preparation time: 15 minutes

Cooking time: 25 minutes

Servings: 8

Ingredients:

Almond flour - ½ cup

Salt - 1 teaspoon

Ground mustard - 1 teaspoon

Black pepper - 1 teaspoon

Xanthan gum - ½ teaspoon

Cayenne pepper - ¼ teaspoon

Heavy cream - ¾ cup

Shredded cheddar cheese - 2 cups

Chopped chives - ¼ cup

Eggs - 6 | Salt - a pinch

Cream of tartar - ¼ teaspoon

Directions:

Preheat your oven at 350 degrees Fahrenheit. Grease your loaf tin.

In a bowl, mix together the almond flour, salt, ground mustard, black pepper, xanthan gum, cayenne pepper with heavy cream and the shredded cheddar cheese.

Now mix in the chopped fresh chives. Make sure that the ingredients are mixed properly.

Separate the egg yolks and the egg whites and mix in the egg yolks in the mixture. In another bowl, beat the egg whites and the cream of tartar until stiff peaks form.

Add a pinch of salt. Fold the egg whites in to the egg yolk mixture to incorporate well.

Pour the mixture in to a greased loaf pan and put them to bake in preheated oven for 20 to 25 minutes or until the bread rises and turns golden brown. Serve hot immediately!

Nutrition:

Calories: 175 | Fats: 9.89 g | Carbs: 10.51 g | Proteins: 9.37 g

GRAIN FREE CASHEW SOURDOUGH BREAD

Preparation time: 30 minutes

Cooking time: 50 minutes

Servings: 12

Ingredients:

Cashews - 10 | Water - 4 ounces

Probiotic capsules - equal to 30-40 billion strains

Eggs, separated - 2 | Water - 1 tablespoon

Baking soda - ½ teaspoon | Salt - ¼ teaspoon

Egg yolk plus water 1 tablespoon

Directions:

Blend the cashews with filtered water. Put the mixture in to a bowl, add in the probiotic capsules and then mix them well.

Cover the bowl and put in the oven which should not be more than 110 degrees for 12 hours at least. The longer you let it sit the more sour it will become.

When it is ready, preheat the oven on 325 degrees. Put the cashew mixture in to a bowl.

Separate both the egg yolks and the egg whites and add the egg yolks in the cashew mixture with the water. Now add the baking soda and salt in the cashew mixture.

Beat the egg whites until soft peaks form and then fold them in the egg yolks and cashew mixture. Pour the mixture in to a prepared loaf tin.

Mix the egg yolk and the water and use the pastry brush for the egg wash.

Bake at 325 degrees for 50 minutes.

Serve when cool.

Nutrition:

Calories: 23 | Fats: 1.62 g | Carbs: 0.49 g | Proteins: 1.5 g

WHOLE WHEAT COCONUT BREAD

Preparation time: 10 minutes

Cooking time: 25 minutes

Servings: 8

Ingredients:

Pastry flour - 1 ½ cups

Sugar - 2 tablespoons

Baking powder - 2 teaspoons

Salt - ½ teaspoon

Milk - 1 ½ cups

Melted coconut oil - 1/3 cup

Egg - 1

Vanilla extract - ½ teaspoon

Directions:

Preheat your oven at 350 degrees Fahrenheit.

Mix together the pastry flour, sugar, baking powder and salt.

Make a well in the center and add in the wet ingredients that are milk, melted coconut oil, egg and vanilla extract.

Pour the batter in to a greased cake pan and cook until the bread turns golden brown for approximately 25 minutes.

Cool and serve!

Nutrition:

Calories: 152 | Fats: 11.98 g | Carbs: 8.72 g | Proteins: 3.03 g

KETO BLUEBERRY LEMON BREAD

Preparation time: 30 minutes

Cooking time: 50 minutes

Servings: 16

Ingredients:

Almond flour - 3 cups

Egg white protein powder - 2 tablespoons

Cream of tartar - 1 teaspoon

Baking soda - ½ teaspoon

Celtic sea salt - ¼ teaspoon

Eggs - 6 | Lemon zest - 1 tablespoon

Vanilla extract - ½ tablespoon

Vanilla stevia - ½ teaspoon

Blue berries - 1 cup

Directions:

In a food processor, blend together the almond flour, egg white protein powder, cream of tartar, baking soda and the salt.

Now add in the eggs, lemon zest, vanilla extract and the vanilla stevia.

Now fold in the blue berries.

Mix the batter well and then pour the batter in to a prepared greased pan.

Preheat your oven at 350 degrees Fahrenheit.

Put the pan to bake in preheated oven for 45 to 50 minutes or until baked to perfection.

Cool and then serve!

Nutrition:

Calories: 85 | Fats: 6.22 g | Carbs: 0.81 g | Proteins: 5.95 g

EASY LOW CARB BAKED BREAD

Preparation time: 15 minutes

Cooking time: 10 minutes

Servings: 12

Ingredients:

Almond flour - 2 ½ cups

Baking powder - 2 teaspoons

Baking soda - ¼ teaspoon

Salt - ¼ teaspoon

Softened butter - ¼ cup

Egg white protein powder - 2 tablespoon

Eggs - 3

Anise extract - 4 teaspoons

Directions:

Preheat your oven at 350 degrees Fahrenheit.

Mix almond flour, baking powder, baking soda and salt in a bowl.

In a separate bowl, beat the butter.

Now add in the eggs, anise extract and beat them with butter.

Now mix in the flour and the egg white protein powder and form the dough.

Cut the dough lengthwise and place the slices on to a prepared baking sheet.

Put the slices to bake in preheated oven for about 10 minutes or until both sides turn brown.

Cool and serve!

Nutrition:

Calories: 75 | Fats: 6.49 g | Carbs: 0.71 g | Proteins: 3.42 g

PROTEIN BREAD

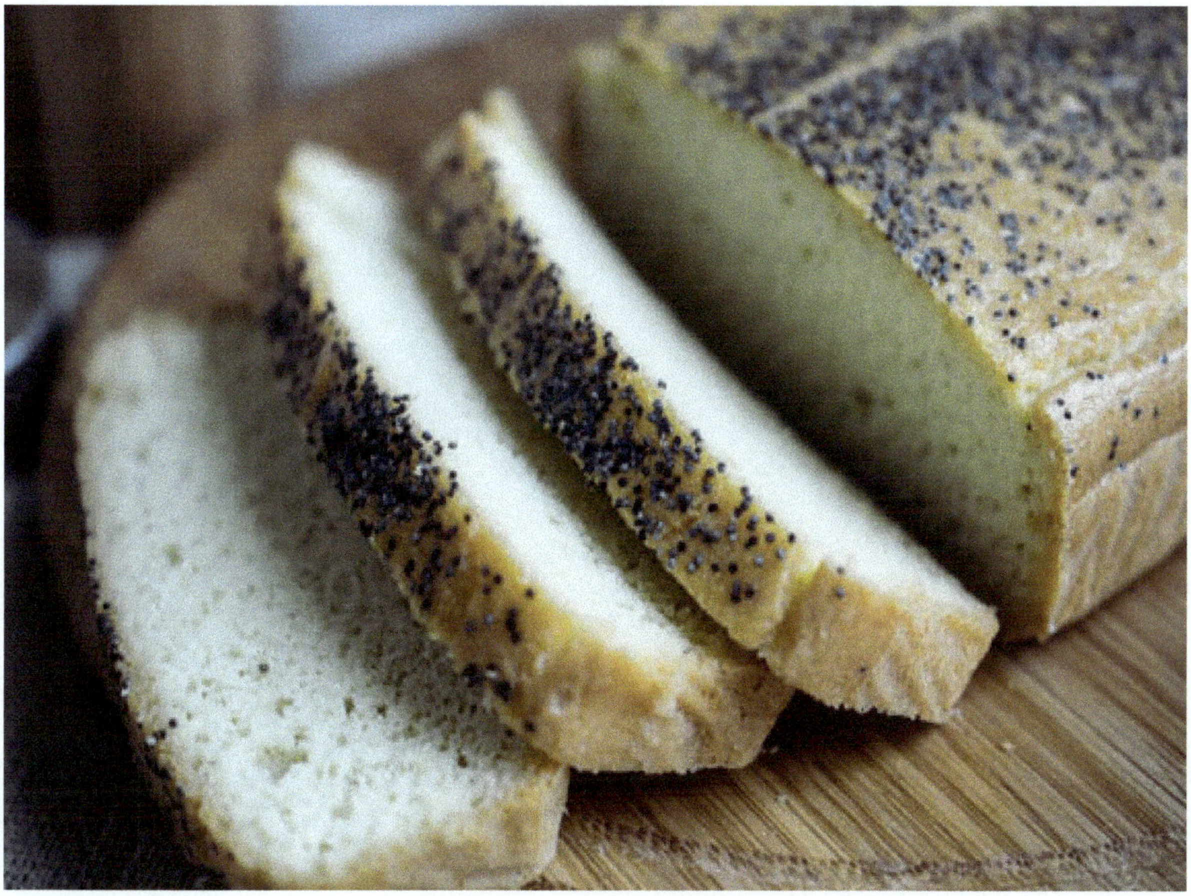

EASY CUCUMBER BREAD

Preparation time: 10 minutes

Cooking time: 50 minutes

Servings: 6

Ingredients:

1 cup erythritol

1 cup coconut oil, melted

1 cup almonds, chopped

1 teaspoon vanilla extract

A pinch of salt

A pinch of nutmeg, ground

½ teaspoon baking powder

A pinch of cloves | 3 eggs

1 teaspoon baking soda

1 tablespoon cinnamon powder

2 cups cucumber, peeled, deseeded and shredded

3 cups coconut flour | Cooking spray

Directions:

In a bowl, mix the flour with cucumber, cinnamon, baking soda, cloves, baking powder, nutmeg, salt, vanilla extract and the almonds and stir well.

Add the rest of the ingredients except the coconut flour, stir well and transfer the dough to a loaf pan greased with cooking spray.

Bake at 325 degrees F for 50 minutes, cool the bread down, slice and serve.

Nutrition:

Calories 243 | Fats 12 g | Fibers 3 g | Carbs 6 g | Proteins 7 g

GREAT BLACKBERRIES BREAD

Preparation time: 10 minutes

Cooking time: 1 hour

Servings: 10

Ingredients:

2 cups almond flour

½ cup stevia

1 and ½ teaspoon baking powder

1 teaspoon baking soda

2 eggs, whisked

1 and ½ cup almond flour

¼ cup ghee, melted

1 tablespoon vanilla extract

1 cup blackberries, mashed

Cooking spray

Directions:

In a bowl, mix the flour with the baking powder, baking soda, stevia, vanilla and blackberries and stir well.

Add the rest of the ingredients, stir the batter and pour it into a loaf pan greased with cooking spray.

Bake at 400 degrees F for 1 hour, cool down, slice and serve.

Nutrition:

Calories 200 | Fats 7 g | Fibers 3 g | Carbs 5 g | Proteins 7 g

KETO RASPBERRIES BREAD

Preparation time: 10 minutes

Cooking time: 50 minutes

Servings: 6

Ingredients:

2 cups almond flour

1 teaspoon baking soda

¾ cup erythritol

A pinch of salt

1 egg

¾ cup coconut milk

¼ cup ghee, melted

2 cups raspberries

2 teaspoons vanilla extract

¼ cup coconut oil, melted

Directions:

In a bowl, mix the flour with the baking soda, erythritol, salt, vanilla and the raspberries and stir.

Add the rest of the ingredients gradually and mix the batter well.

Pour this into a lined loaf pan and bake at 350 degrees F for 50 minutes.

Cool the bread down, slice and serve.

Nutrition:

Calories 200 | Fats 7 g | Fibers 3 g | Carbs 5 g | Proteins 7 g

LOW CARB YEAST BREAD

Preparation time: 10 minutes

Cooking time: 4 hours

Servings: 16 slices

Ingredients :

1 teaspoon salt

4 tablespoons oat flour

1 package dry yeast rapid rise/highly active

1 1/2 teaspoons baking powder

1/2 teaspoon sugar

1 1/8 cups warm water

1/4 cup coarse unprocessed wheat bran

3 tablespoons olive oil

1/4 cup flax meal

1 cup vital wheat gluten flour

3/4 cup soy flour

Directions:

Add water, yeast and sugar to the bread machine and let rest there for 10 minutes.

Add the remaining ingredients and select bread mode on the machine.

After the cooking time is over, remove the bread from the machine and let rest for about 10 minutes. Enjoy!

Nutrition:

Calories 99 | Fats 5 g | Total Carbs 7 g | Proteins 9 g

SEEDED BREAD

Preparation time: 10 minutes

Cooking time: 40 minutes

Servings: 16 slices

Ingredients :

2 tablespoons chia seeds

1/4 teaspoon salt

7 large eggs

1/2 teaspoon xanthan gum

2 cups almond flour

1 teaspoon baking powder

1/2 cup unsalted butter

3 tablespoons sesame seeds

2 tablespoons olive oil

Directions:

Add all the ingredients to the bread machine.

Close the lid and choose bread mode.

Once done, take out from machine and cut into at least 16 slices.

This keto seeded bread can be kept for up to 4-5 days in the fridge.

Nutrition:

Calories 101 | Fats 16 g | Total Carbs 4 g | Proteins 6 g

CINNAMON SWEET BREAD

Preparation time: 10 minutes

Cooking time: 1 hour

Servings: 12

Ingredients :

3 teaspoons ground cinnamon

1 ½ cups of almond flour

3 large eggs

½ cup keto sweetener

1 teaspoon vanilla essence

¼ cup coconut flour

¼ cup sour cream

1 teaspoon baking powder

½ cup unsweetened almond milk

½ cup unsalted butter, melted

Directions:

Add all ingredients to the bread machine.

Close the lid and choose the sweet bread mode.

After the cooking time is over, remove the bread from the machine and let rest for about 10 minutes. Enjoy!

Nutrition:

Calories 191 | Fats 17 g | Total Carbs 5 g | Proteins 5 g

NUT AND SEED BREAD

Preparation time: 35 minutes

Cooking time: 45 minutes

Servings: 16 slices

Ingredients :

1 cup pumpkin seeds

1 teaspoon salt

1/2 cup almond flour

4 eggs, whisked

1/2 cup whole almonds

1 tablespoon lemon juice

1 cup raw pecans

¼ cup olive oil

1/2 cup hazelnuts

1/4 cup poppy seeds

1/2 cup flax meal

1 cup sunflower seeds

1/2 cup chia seeds

Directions:

Add all the ingredients to the bread machine.

Close the lid and choose bread mode.

Once done, take out from machine and cut into at least 16 slices.

Nutrition:

Calories 316 | Fats 28 g | Total Carbs 11 g | Proteins 11 g

ALMOND BREAD LOAF

Preparation time: 10 minutes

Cooking time: 3 hours and 22 minutes

Servings: 15

Ingredients:

2 ½ cups almond flour

1/3 cup coconut flour

½ teaspoon xanthan gum

1 ½ teaspoons baking powder

¼ teaspoon salt Sesame seeds

¼ cup butter, melted and cooled

5 eggs

2/3 cup almond milk

¼ teaspoon tartar cream

Directions:

Add all the ingredients to the bread machine.

Close the lid and choose bread mode.

Once done, take out from machine and cut into at least 16 slices.

Nutrition:

Calories 215 | Fats 10.1 g | Total Carbs 5 g | Proteins 25.2 g

SUGAR FREE BANANA BREAD

Preparation time: 10 minutes

Cooking time: 3 hours and 18 minutes

Servings: 8

Ingredients:

1 ½ cups almond flour

¼ cup granulated erythritol sweetener

1 teaspoon baking powder

2 teaspoons cinnamon

¼ cup walnuts, crushed

½ cup banana, mashed

2 tablespoons butter, melted

3 eggs

Directions:

Add all ingredients to the bread machine.

Close the lid and choose the sweet bread mode.

After the cooking time is over, remove the bread from the machine and let rest for about 10 minutes. Enjoy!

Nutrition:

Calories 205 | Fats 17.2 g | Total Carbs 6.4 g | Proteins 8 g

CONCLUSION

Keto bread is not just another keto recipe. It's a balanced low carb bread that can be used as a meal replacement.Each of the issues is a suggestion that your body is in ketosis.

These are a few of the signs you will observe as you begin the transition:

You may experience keto flu or induction flu, which includes let down mental functions and energy. You may suffer from sleeping problems, bouts of nausea, augmented hunger, or other possible gastrointestinal worries. Several days into the keto plan should remedy these effects. If not, add ½ of a teaspoon of salt into a glass of water and drink it to help with the side effects. For the first week, you may need to do this daily. It could take up to 15 to 20 minutes before it helps. It will improve with time.

You may also notice an aroma similar to nail polish. Not surprising because this is acetone, a ketone product. It may also give you a unique body odor as your body adjusts to the diet changes. Maintain good oral health and use a breath refresher if needed.

Leg cramps may be an issue as you begin ketosis. The loss of magnesium (a mineral) can be a demon and create a bit of pain with the onset of the keto diet plan changes. With the loss of the minerals during urination, you could experience bouts of cramps in your legs.

Of course, the keto diet also has benefits that include:

Remain Satiated: Fat and protein are more filling and will stick to your ribs longer than products that are occupied with carbohydrates.

Dravet Syndrome: Dravet Syndrome is a severe form of epilepsy marked by prolonged, uncontrollable, and frequent seizures, which began in infancy. Unfortunately, available medications don't improve symptoms in approximately one-third of the Dravet Syndrome patients.

A clinical study used 13 children with Dravet Syndrome to stay on the ketogenic diet for more than one year to remain seizure-free. Over 50% of the group decreased in the frequency of the seizures. Six of the patients stopped the diet later, and one remains seizure-free.

Mental Focus: Your brain is approximately 60% fat by weight. By increasing your fatty food intake, you will have a better focus. It can maintain itself and work at total capacity.

Blood Pressure Levels Lowered: When you begin the ketogenic diet, your blood pressure may become lower, making you feel dizzy at first. Don't worry or feel overly concerned because that's a clear indication that the carbohydrates are working. However, if you are currently taking medications, it's a good idea to speak with your physician about the possibility of lowering some of your doses while on the ketogenic or intermittent fasting plan.

Polycystic Ovary Syndrome (PCOS): Young women of childbearing years can be affected by this disorder. It is further also associated with obesity, insulin resistance, and hyperinsulinemia. One study concluded a significant improvement in weight loss in fasting women over 24-weeks. The group limited carb intake to 20 grams daily for 24 weeks, which led to its success.

There are many more benefits, but you now have a good idea of how much better you can feel if you follow the keto techniques of dieting.

CPSIA information can be obtained
at www.ICGtesting.com
Printed in the USA
LVHW061137130422
716028LV00008B/453